Dr George William Bryan is a retired child psychiatrist living in the suburbs of Paris, France, with his wife Genevieve. He has practiced psychiatry in the suburbs of Los Angeles, California, specializing in adolescent juvenile offenders, with training in psychoanalytic theory. His first wife died several years ago after a protracted illness, resulting in his turning to a different view of what he had been writing for many years. This tragedy, along with his meditation, led to a spiritual awakening that resulted in his pursuit of ethereal variables entwined in our psychological makeup. His first work, *Reflections on Us*, explored the personal elements of this, with the present book emphasizing the psychological and spiritual interplay within all of us.

To Genevieve, my window to Heaven.

George William Bryan

THE MYSTERY OF US

AUSTIN MACAULEY PUBLISHERS™

LONDON • CAMBRIDGE • NEW YORK • SHARJAH

A CIP catalogue record for this title is available from the British Library.

ISBN 9781398436688 (Paperback)
ISBN 9781398436695 (ePub e-book)

www.austinmacauley.com

First Published 2022
Austin Macauley Publishers Ltd®
1 Canada Square
Canary Wharf
London
E14 5AA

I acknowledge all who had the insight to see the other, more than themselves, and the capacity to communicate themselves to the other.

Table of Contents

Preface

This volume is a collection of verses that reflect the pursuit of personal, inner phenomenology, as well as reflections on our psychological make-up. While easily read, the occasional rereading of selections may reward the inquisitive reader of multiple meanings that may have heuristic value for them. It is hoped that this preface will enhance some clarification and understanding prior to, or after, they have been read.

The formal religions offer strength personally, as well as through community involvement. They all have their own structure and dogma. Within each of us is a religious sentiment, as noted by William James, that is deeply personal and may, or may not, be connected to a formal religion. It is to that personal religious sentiment that most of these verses are directed, and all of them are relevant to our psychological make-up. So, the verses do not reflect any specific religion as such, but rather express the experiences and feelings of the individual seeker. In other words, they pursue questions we all ask ourselves at various moments in our lives, and some, with a whisper, offer a hint of an answer.

In the first volume I underscored personal experiences, with elements of psychological knowledge. In this volume much the same is continued but with greater emphasis on the interplay of the psychological and the spiritual. There is a continued emphasis on the anxiety-relieving qualities noted through the sense of being emotionally connected, be it in a relationship with an individual, in a group, with pets, through material substances like books, or with a perceived deity. This reflects elements of the psychoanalyst, Heinz Kohut, and his school of thought referred to as Self Psychology. I do not believe that he ever pursued the specific phenomenon of the religious, but his thoughts appear easily applicable to that pursuit and the hope is that my utilising them in that context will not be cause for offence to his followers.

Personally, I remain struck, and frankly awed, by the power of experiencing the wonder, and Love of a "Higher Power". Is this psychological? Of course. Is it a function of imagination, illusion? Perhaps, but not necessarily. There appears no easy explanation except to those who are dogmatic, or offended. Certainly, there exist phenomenology that are not easily explained.

Carl Jung attempted explanations through his concept of the Collective Unconscious. Sigmund Freud wrote them off as illusory, neurotic, or even psychotic, such as drug-induced. Individuals will follow what makes sense to them. Our inner world remains essentially accessible to the individual alone and can be explored by only that individual. Obviously reporting experiences to others, and/or utilising machines such as an MRI can help, but science remains strongest and most credible exploring the outside world, not our inner experiences. William James had the capacity to be open to this without histrionic declarations, nor rigid denials. He acknowledged that there appeared to be phenomenology not explained by our philosophy or science. The verses reflect my personal experiences and the careful reader will hopefully have a sense of this, as they represent an attempt to communicate the non-verbal through the media of poetry.

Jung attempted to bridge the world of common experience to that of personal inner reflection, and the treasured sense of the numinous. At the end of his life he stated regretting not succeeding in conveying the reality that humans have souls. These verses are an attempt to share that reality in a manner comfortable to receive, and evocative enough to encourage others to seek inner experiences and convictions.

We are conscious, intelligent creatures that, in a sense, sit on an evolved animal brute. This fact has been symbolised in mythology and utilised as a metaphor by Freud regarding sitting on a horse, the horse being the view of his concept of the Id. Our culture is an evolved machination of our consciousness and intellect, tending to colour this fact of our biology. Evolution has favoured the animal of us with selective emphasis on competitiveness, aggressiveness, sexuality, and animal bonding. These also being counterbalanced and modified by our intellect and adaptive mores. Nonetheless, the animal of us continues to be insidious, bothersome, or dominant depending upon the individual, pathology, or uncontrollable events. All of this is reflected in many of the verses.

Both Freud and Jung emphasised the presence in us of the unconscious. That when it is made conscious it allows for control of elements of earlier traumas, as well as for qualities of our more bestial potentials, or even numinous, or spiritual experiences. To remain unconscious can result in maladaptation, the most common being that of projection. Projection is the psychological mechanism of attributing your unconscious impulses or qualities as coming from another source in the outside world and denying that they exist within one's self. Another way of saying this is that your "demons", so to speak, are seen as coming at you instead of from you. Jung believed that our tendency to deal with our unconscious by projection was common, and an explanation of much of our social problems. Freud was less impressed by this dynamic, but concurred with projection being a bothersome psychological defence.

Comment is offered on the issue of "social engineering", which in and of itself appears to be a noble endeavour, but tends to devalue the religious, as well as valuing the collective over the individual. I must admit to bias because of my emphasis on the individual and the individual's task of personal advancement psychologically and spiritually, and suspicious of solutions that have a collective, or "external" orientation. Frequently collective plans are twisted, because of zeal, to coercive solutions, that impinge upon the independence of individuals. It is the old cliché of, "be careful of those who insist that they know what's best for you". Also, it is my conviction that it is our inner world where reality is found, and the outer experiences are but manifestations of our inner interpretations. Significant world changes occur when this is acknowledged, which is a characteristic of viable world religions, that underscore the individual's task of religious humility and gives credence to personal religious practice and experiences. Social engineering, instead, underscores collective manipulation and pursuing measures that "are for the good of society" at large. This hints at impatience at best, and ambitions of power at worse. I have found that the religious sentiment mentioned by James appears to be present in us all, but is manifest in a variety of ways. In the personal experience it clearly is profound and awe inspiring, but when turned to others it can become distorted and silly. Thus, while quite different philosophically, John Dewey and Karl Marx both hoped for humanity to achieve a heaven on earth, which is marginally absurd when one realises that we struggle with millions of years of evolutionary debris where the genetically successful sit on top of the shredded flesh and bones of the "losers". The animal of us is both ubiquitous and powerful, so what is the answer to its hold on us? …….See it. Have the humility to acknowledge its presence. You see it in dreams, in fantasy, music and art preferences, and thoughts. Also, take care regarding what is found most repulsive or horrifying, as the unconscious is tricky, and what may appear most repulsive in fact might be the opposite in your depths. Know well researched history, as it is filled with examples of foolish pursuits of power, greed, aggression, etc., frequently justified as noble, or even "spiritually" driven, or "for the betterment of mankind". I do not know if we can collectively succeed, but I do know that we can individually succeed. That is the point of these verses.

As noted above, the importance of feeling connected emotionally is also recognised. I believe that it was the psychoanalyst, Donald Winnicott, who put forth the idea of "ego relatedness", which is the state of emotional connection between individuals without the elements of cognitive qualities which would be found in psychoanalytic transference reactions. To facilitate easier understanding the term "connection" is utilised in all of the verses instead of that of "ego relatedness", or that of "empathy". Heinz Kohut underscored this dynamic, as well as the consequences of it not occurring. He pointed out the example of the infant/mother-figure bonding, and how this generalises outwardly to others, as well as to objects (such as "the teddy bear"). Thus, feeling connected is thought to be imperative for emotional health. The richer our psychological connections, the greater the control over the animal. The opposite is also true, the less our psychological connecting the greater power of the animal (I refer the reader to the anecdotes of the abandoned child, regarding India's « Wolf Boy »). This is also reflected in our tendency to idealise or sacrifice our individuality in the service of some group or community. A positive or negative consequence is readily seen in military organisations, or in various social movements. There is no question as to the uplifting experience of sensing a connection with the infinite. This may be understood through the various views noted above.

Finally, there is the phenomena of annihilation anxiety which is a consequence of experiencing a sense of profound disconnection or feeling totally overwhelmed. For Kohut, this is ameliorated through the process of connecting emotionally. In the adult this may be understood as a regression back to the emotional state of the infant's total helplessness. But for the adult who experiences a sense of being held, or uplifted, is this simply a "regression"? Or is it a phenomenology in the realm of the numinous? This is explored at length in these verses.

Whether one pursues therapy, contemplation, learning to understand one's dreams, gardening, humble prayer, etc., the point is to underscore inner experiences as frequently as comfortable. As you do so, with patience, it will be found to offer comfort, a growth in perspective, a feeling of ease, and a growing sense of gratitude. Love appears to be present the deeper one pursues the inner depths of self. Acceptance of a "Higher Power" also presents itself to you, which appears to be associated with an increasing sense of humility. Jung alludes to this in his works on the collective unconscious and the archetypes. All of which is fine reading, but the essence of one's pursuit is your personal experience. This is reflected in many of the verses.

I am brought back to the wonder of experiencing the feeling of pervasive, infusing love that is without verbal comprehension. I have attempted to communicate this throughout many of these verses, as well as underscoring of the insidious presence of primitive elements within us. This struggle that we all have with our evolutionary roots and our use of the newly achieved quality of consciousness to reach for something beyond it, is a constant theme. Again, the hope is that the verses will evoke the sense of the numinous, the reality of having a soul, and encourage others to be comfortable pursuing their inner experiences. Most importantly, with all the experts milling about in our world, the single most perceptive expert of you, will always remain, simply, ……. you.

An Introduction

I can denigrate my senses,
I can denigrate my thoughts,
I can denigrate experience,
Or can, of course, choose not.

Thus is nature of free will,
An asset of our consciousness.
Contributes to the sense of guilt,
But also to inventiveness.

Sincerity's important too,
Attempting to be clear.
Discarding what's illusory,
Holding what is dear.

As critics tend to emphasise,
Subjective is suspect.
Objective more reliable,
Engenders shared respect.

The problem remains obvious,
Introspection weak.
The personal so powerful,
But sharing out of reach.

Remaining with a cautious tone,
Critical and clear.
Choosing a poetic style,
To share what is sincere.

What's offered as an easy read,
Will deepen if persist.
And leave you, with a gentleness,
That spirit does exist.

Science scoffs by inference,
Try never to forget.
Be confident as peer in deep,
Your evidence direct.

To John S. Peck, Md, PhD

It never ceases to amaze me,
To exist in life of ours.
Flying through this sense of time,
Passing all these hours.

Reflecting as I do this moment
Writing what are lines.
Entertaining deep pretensions,
Animal maligns.

Consciousness and intellect,
Convey a sense profound.
When in fact, truth be said,
It's mostly empty ground.

We operate with high intent,
To reach the stars beyond.
Rushing to increase control,
Not breaking free of bond.

Eat the fruit, as wait to fall,
A Zen approach at best.
Hide despair, put forth a smile,
Await to be at rest.

Is it all for nothing,
This life that we endure?
Seeking to find meaning,
In all that is explored?

Can elevate the memory
Of those that are no more.
It's kind of like an honour,
As they no longer soar.

Clearly it's the living,
Pay homage with respect,
To those who have affected us,
Have taught us to connect.

In all that we do elevate,
Of lives that aren't misleading
The ones with whom we idolise
Hint at life's true meaning.

Their capacity to empathize,
Acts as guide to all.
Teaching a connection,
A model to recall.

As we grieve what has been lost,
The animal is gone.
Their spirit that reflects their life,
Gives clue where we belong.

If only see the animal
The lesson is obscured.
Instead find what is spirit,
Implicit as the cure.

Through living life's long journey,
Recognising Truth.
It's care and Love's connecting,
We honour as its root.

William James

Here's a read,
For those so inclined,
The Father of American Psychology.

William James, a man to respect.
Had the ability with care to instruct.
Strict in his science, perceptive in thought,
Balanced and clear when in darkness he walked.

Able to question illusion and hope,
Not be entangled with magic and smoke.
Yet open in mind, not conditioned and tight,
Aware of the mystery found in this life.

Power of culture to blind and confuse,
We eat and we breath it, within it's infused.
Creates preconceptions, convictions alike,
Closing the mind, creating our night.

This can be true of religious or not,
Dogma and bias controlling our thought.
Thus those like James, important to know,
Free-thinking and open a gift is bestowed.

Both Freud and Jung together agreed,
Regarding his exceptionality.
Freud impressed at his endurance,
And Jung with his mentality.

The Mystery of Us

Cannot escape the obvious,
As look around at life.
It's varied and miraculous,
A clear earthly delight.

The miracle it hints at,
Even science would agree,
Keeps the head a spinning,
Humbling all who simply see.

As deep as one may peer,
Or thoughtful reverie,
The order it does manifest,
Leaves clear a mystery.

Watch the birthing of the young,
Or growth from tiny seeds,
Staggers the imagining,
Makes small our sense of being.

If pause a bit, simply marvel,
The wonder of it all.
Surely over-powering
An answer we recall.

Having the ability
To slow, and take it in,
Can leave one with amazement,
To all that is and been.

Not to have the skill
Of a William Blake,
Doesn't alter mystery
Of nature we partake.

Simply left to share with all,
Despite how much we know.
Nature is enigma,
With spirit undisclosed.

Jung's View

Jung discovered a world
That belongs to all of us.
A world within, of good and evil,
As well as rage and lust.

So deep it lies, cannot perceive,
A record of our eons.
Archives of the distant past,
Prior to our being.

He suspected energies
Affect us every day.
Some are viewed as archetypes,
It's dreams where they display.

He called this the Unconscious,
The Collective to be clear.
Unlike Freud's repression,
It isn't singular.

What makes his thought of careful note,
His conviction that is stressed,
The amazing power in us all,
Of pious, with the blasphemous.

Because of evolution's stroke,
Selection is ascendant.
But with advent of consciousness,
Religious is transcendent.

He posits we have Deity
Within, awaiting notice.
But we also have selection's host
A myriad to goad us.

We have a lengthy past,
But a sacred acquisition.
A never-ending task,
To reach for intercession.

Projection

Fantasies enrich our lives,
But also cause us grief.
A variation on the thoughts
That spin without relief.

Thinking is incessant,
At all levels of the mind.
They're the root of shame and doubt,
Preventing the sublime.

To complicate this process,
Is with ease that we project.
Projection is our tendency
Throw out, as self-protect.

All of this makes primitive,
Interactions one might have.
Underscores awareness,
As a goal that's not so bad.

To look within, or pause a bit,
More clear to see one's self.
Increase aware of who you are,
See other with less filth.

Such the nature of us beings,
For better or for worse.
It works best for us when seeing
Our primate and its curse.

Psychoanalysis

Psychoanalysis, as taught by Freud,
A boon to who you are.
Helping one to clarify
A painful childhood scar.

But when complete, the task persists,
As an inner view suggested.
Knowing where you come from,
More than animal invested.

Awareness of connections
That highlight genealogy.
Turning deep attention
To questions of theology.

Seems we tend to idolise
The various and the sundry.
Always raising questions
Of seeking what might One be.

The idealising process
Can involve the group one's in.
If lose attention to one's self
Illusion can begin.

When this happens strength is felt,
But only with the group.
You as individual,
Lost within the loop.

Believing one has answers,
Questions cease to be.
What may be a Reality
With mockery we flee

Continued self-analysis,
Explore with growing patience.
Find an increased clarity
Of sacred in existence.

Note as ideals fall away,
A single One is found.
The sense to be uplifted,
Your clue of what is sound.

This to simply try to state:
Once clear of your biology,
The sacred plain of consciousness,
Jung searched as a psychology.

Holy Grail

In the past,
Was pursuit, of the Holy Grail.
At the time,
Was thought, to be quite real.

Knights of old would search for it,
Difficult to find.
Because was not objectified,
The goal a different kind.

Something sacred, held so dear,
Search tenaciously.
Unaware it found so near,
A singularity.

Alchemists then underscored
A Stone of precious power.
Also found the rung too high,
A reach with constant flounder.

Now we enter the mind's space,
With thought that never ceases.
Still searching for what is divine,
Mathematics is our thesis.

Instead of what was holy,
We reach to know it all.
Expanding how we find ourselves,
Pulled on by Siren's call.

Focus seems upon us,
Our primate crows with pride.
We've lost pursuit of Maker,
Instead alone we stride.

Yet, pause so ever briefly,
Look in, instead of out,
Recover sense of smallness,
In a universe devout.

To do so holds perspective,
For the animal of us.
Allowing for our spirit,
To flourish, not be hushed.

What has endlessly been searched for,
Begins to lift its veil.
With gratitude on finding,
In you, the Holy Grail.

Ubiquitous Fancy

Why do fantasies enthral us so?
As if our thoughts are all we know.
Such power seems to dominate,
View of life invigorate.

If such fancy were to mute,
Tempered down a bit.
How would life appear to us,
Duller perhaps a whit?

They range from full adventure,
To simple slips of dreams.
Entangle those we're close to,
Within our private themes.

Not rarely do they dictate
Our take on one another.
Frequent casting shadow,
As Real is darkly covered.

You see this in relationships,
That seem to go awry.
But even in successful ones
Imaginings still thrive.

With discipline, is found the arts,
And science at its best.
Still, if pause to listen,
There is wildness when at rest.

A different possibility,
As thought is everywhere,
We truly are the primate,
With thinking our despair.

Question remains present,
Still not very clear,
What is found if thinking
Was to cease its constant blare.

It seems when thought
Is minimised, or more,
One finds a blush of gratitude,
A wonder to explore.

Instead of constant fantasy,
Or calculated musing.
The warmth of Love expansive,
With One who is infusing.

But holding such a wonder,
Is difficult to do.
Thoughts are dominating,
They own us through and through.

Perhaps to know the moments,
Of gratitude and Love,
Helps to keep attention,
To the Mystery Above.

The Primitive Within

The primate, that is us,
Is a subtle navigator.
We notice not its presence,
Deceives as instigator.

Whether work, and then at play,
Its presence is our shadow.
Because we have a rush of thoughts,
Stays hidden in the babel.

Eons it has thrived alone,
Only recent we ascended.
Sitting high upon our throne,
When noted, feel offended.

Yet its power, quite a fright,
Controls us without notice.
Uses all our new found tools,
With beastly different focus.

Evolution taught it strength,
Control, and domination.
Such goals remain, in spite of speech,
Can lead to degradation.

As bluster, or coerce another,
Its presence is quite clear.
But presenting logic argument,
Can disguise, and not appear.

What is called progressive,
In fact, may only be,
A clever, dressed up primate,
Intentions shadowy.

The counterpoise of primitive,
Occurs when look within.
Finding hint of gratitude,
Is where you can begin.

Letting go, and opening,
Attend to what's Above.
Imbues the self with thankfulness,
And growing sense of Love.

Science

Brief the time of science,
Dizzy its achievements.
Humbling the review of it,
Amazing in its keenness.

It's not the scientific thought,
Not how far we've come,
But making it a deity,
Our spirit over-run.

When marvel at its history,
The fight to overcome,
Rigid theologic views,
Dogma to be numbed.

Now it seems we've made a turn,
From religious rigid thought,
To that of science attitude,
The sacred being scoffed.

Positivists lead the way,
The real is that of senses.
Negating intuitions sway,
Not measurement intensive.

An irony presents itself,
As humans gain in power.
Diminishing the singular,
Collective builds its Tower.

The irony is simply said,
What's real is deeply personal.
A consciousness within the head,
Is you, and not dispersible.

Again, the wonder that is science,
A treasure to respect.
But finding your religious sense,
A gift to not neglect.

Can't be measured or controlled,
A particular experience.
The source of it is very old,
Gentle yet Imperious.

Prison of Thought

Here's a thought, no need for more,
A paradox is present.
It's thinking that prevents the Real,
From showing its true essence.

Thinking is a useful tool,
But we use it to our harm.
In science, math, philosophy
It works just like a charm.

But notice how it dominates,
Fills our minds with piffle.
From fantasies, imaginings,
To rank and ugly drivel.

It seems in sacred places,
Or anywhere at all,
Our thoughts just keep on wandering
On something's beck and call.

Whether you psychologise,
Or offer something clever,
It remains a simple fact to note,
Our thoughts appear forever!

But if you find a time to pause,
A space between each thought,
You begin to sense a freeing up,
A move to what is sought.

When looking for that free space,
The sense of looking in,
Attention to this inner self
Allows you to begin.

Call it meditation,
Or perhaps, a simple prayer,
Finding in thought's absence,
Reality 'comes clear.

The process does take patience,
But with hope, one does succeed.
The specialness of you is clear,
Allow this to be freed.

The Soul Within

As the body ages,
Or begins to run its course.
One can find self-roaring,
Until the voice is hoarse.

Of course it all means nothing,
Genetics rule the day.
We ride along oblivious,
At end we start to bay.

Complaining seems ubiquitous,
A puzzle in a sense.
Appears most are insensitive
Can only see their fence.

It takes some time, and maybe trust,
Whatever, it's a task.
But inward turning carefully,
Will help in, awareness.

Much of life is spent in fear,
Hidden from clear view.
The primate that has always been,
Driving much of you.

As it ages, slowing down,
The time is ripe to see.
A crystal sense of who you are,
A soul, through all eternity.

The Ordinary

When a mystery is solved,
There's little interest left.
It takes away the energy
From what was full of zest.

Imaginings feed mystery
With questions and the like.
There's wonder and excitement,
The darker is the night.

But finding fancy weakened,
With explanations clear,
May offer some assurance,
But lessens what is dear.

There really is a question
Of the origin of us.
The numinous phenomena,
Leads to thoughtfulness.

In wonder at existing,
As primates, we observe.
Try to lift above us,
But drop into the herd.

Like all the other animals
Hardwired we exist.
Doing what is programmed,
Still, wilfulness persists.

The will, to look in deeper,
To see with clearer view.
May find a sense transcendent,
And Love that reflects You.

Simian

Every now and then,
At moments unexpected,
A sense of something sinister
Seems lurking, not suspected.

It appears this not unusual,
We all possess this darkness,
It's just that when it does occur,
Unsettling, in its starkness.

Contemplate its origin?
Demonic? Or innate?
Makes no difference in the end,
We're all, at root, an ape.

Work so hard to hide this fact,
With pomp and ceremony.
But watch the great, with careful eye,
You'll find what might be phony.

It's not something to hide with shame,
Instead, acknowledge, self-awareness.
The seeing this that's deep within,
Allows control, in all its bareness.

The hiding that we struggle with,
Causes much of grief.
Projecting it on others,
Act out to find relief.

If able to accept the dark,
Not act on evil thinking.
Find the pause between each thought,
To reach for what you're seeking.

It's aloneness and the pain of this
That pulls us down to evil.
The counter to the animal,
Is Love's animus upheaval.

Grace

I passed a man, a boy?
As walking near the Seine.
He appeared in full despondency,
His head in hands, dismayed.

Quietly he sat,
Eyes hidden in his fists.
Never did he move,
As if to not exist.

This life we all do live,
Amazing as it flows,
But for some it is a misery,
A waste that Heaven knows.

Of course there is the need to help,
For those caught in despair.
Still, got me to be thinking,
Why him, not me, who cared?

Expression used too easily,
"There but for God's Grace…"
Wonder at events in past,
Good fortune? Luck? Or Fate?

Always comes to settle back,
With loving gratitude,
Aware a Hand is gently there,
Not seen, or felt, but True.

Gift of Awareness

The body is a tool we use,
Very much like thought.
It's useful to attentive be,
If control is what is sought.

Can signal through emotions,
Or sensations that are raw.
We all are simply primates,
But can learn its early call.

The gift of our awareness
Offers tool to self-explore.
In doing so may pause a bit,
To thank our Maker for.

Whatever view one has of this,
A fact remains as true.
Aware of self and body,
Is indeed a sacred view.

Aphorisms

"Life isn't where you go, it's where you are."
So deep are aphorisms.
It's always hoped the author
Has a modicum of wisdom.

Jewels of expression
In words that seem to scintillate.
Derived from constant thinking,
Some even can illuminate.

The wisdom is simplicity,
From the density of chaos.
Finding what is singular
In what had been a morass.

Of interest in this life of ours
Is thinking, ever present.
Some have skill in thinning it,
To make it more significant.

Thus thinking is a useful tool,
To clarify confusion.
But seeking what is numinous,
Can lead you to illusion.

Finding space in cluttered time,
To pause and be within.
A quiet prayer or emptiness
Helps you to transcend.

So enjoy the clever sayings,
The fruit of focused minds.
But recognise the task to stop
Attention to what binds.

In you, is where you're seeking.
Within, is where you'll find,
A quiet place to rest in,
The shrine of the Divine.

Beyond Material

The body slowly does decay
Consciousness watches, in dismay.
That's the price of entropy,
It's how the body's made.

Now a question might arise,
Am I stuck in body's fate?
Are we left to temporise,
As await to dissipate?

Belief appears as scientific,
Has many answers, viewed terrific.
Sees our life, deep and boldly,
Explores genetics clear but coldly.

Its answers thin when body dies,
The interest seems to wane.
The mystic offers answers,
But appear, alas, inane.

Again the question does occur,
In this universe, are we but chance?
As we sense the world around us,
Do we miss the subtle glance?

Is there something judging us,
That is senseless to our thinking?
In ways beyond our rationale,
Is there Love that is unblinking?

Questions turn without fatigue,
Our thoughts just keep on thinking.
If find a moment where there's pause,
Intuit what you're seeking.

It's there in quiet gratitude,
A growth of something more.
Have trust in what is ill-defined,
Your soul, with Love, will soar.

A Different View

In the world of finite,
Time is always king.
It dictates all decisions,
Permeates our being.

Life and death surround us,
As token of its power.
It runs us like a current,
Can take us any hour.

The mate of it is entropy,
Another to despair.
Together they rule all of us,
Imprisoned in their lair.

Science works to overcome
The power they present.
But will admit that in the end
Both overwhelm our wit.

All this is to focus on
The universe at large.
Atom and its energy,
Material in charge.

But pause a bit and look within,
Find a different space.
A timeless sense, no thought to stir,
A peaceful, soft embrace.

Perhaps this is simplistic,
With logic minimised.
But turn attention inward
And find self-maximised.

The world is seen subjective,
Moist in its perception.
Objective is a dead place,
Dry in its reception.

Have Faith in what's beyond us,
With open heart and yearning.
Quietly receptive,
Grateful for the caring.

Identification

When identify with one group,
To find out who you are.
It helps one to feel special,
But can lead you too afar.

Us humans are the same,
Except for surface shade.
A mix of ape and spirit,
It's how that we were made.

The spirit is quite subtle,
Except for consciousness.
The primate that we're mixed with,
Stirs much that is amiss.

Science studies well
The material and the genes.
But in the realm of numinous
Its tools are much too lean.

So what are you to reach for,
Who to seek to be?
Might turn to one's Creator,
Beware of forgery.

Grieving

When you find yourself with loss,
An emptiness to bear,
It's the animal adapting to
A space within its lair.

Grief, with thoughts, envelope you,
A pain too sharp to hold.
The animal is struggling,
As it has since days of old.

It's difficult, exhausting,
When grasping for control.
The simian keeps screaming,
And ruminations roll.

Thinking is futility,
Persists in senseless ways.
Abortive cogitating,
Prolongs your ailing days.

Try to have attention
Within, an upward reach.
Turn from creature's raging,
In hope, you may beseech.

With humble supplication,
Away from jaws efface,
Whisper, soft and tender,
Hints a Loving firm embrace.

Perspective grows, with gratitude,
Find you're not alone.
A growing sense, with tearfulness,
He's there, above the gloom.

Beneath Illusion

Here's a view to understand,
The you, who well you are.
Not pleasant, but important,
To know the us, below the bar.

It's dissolution terror,
We all do struggle with.
Not felt as such, hides from view,
A crumbling monolith.

Diversion is the game,
That we all use to avoid.
Run as fast as possible,
Just make a lot of noise.

When slow the pace,
A numbing does appear.
The quality of boredom,
Pervasive with a leer.

There is apparent irony,
As sink into this core.
It's alive with painful terror,
Not dead as was before.

Despair does slowly creep in,
As you struggle with the Real.
It's here that self-destruction,
As an option, you can feel.

But have a Faith to hold you,
Or hope, to drive you on.
Begin to find a settling,
A growing glow beyond.

It's here a sense of gratitude,
Meld's gently with Love's sway.
A subtle note you're not alone,
No matter if it's vague.

Beauty of Love

Boundaries are important
To know from whence we came.
Unless you are a Buddhist,
Believe we're all the same.

Now I know it's hard on Buddhists,
Who insist nirvana vague,
The oceanic feeling,
A Freudian might say.

To stand alone is frightening,
But it's really all we are.
The value of the other,
Helps see what is afar.

When love occurs,
Magic is perceived.
Sense engulfed by beauty,
As if returned to Eve.

All these views important,
To peruse and understand.
But turn to your experience,
From there to take a stand.

When experts say we all are one,
Wonder if what's meant,
We all are what the expert is?
Controls environment?

Feeling you are well again,
No longer all alone.
It's love that brings you to that point,
A sense of being home.

As life draws on, events occur,
Distance from each other.
Causing sense of meaningless,
When it's love that's gone asunder.

A singular in multiple,
Enhanced by love's embrace.
From relationship with one held dear,
To ascendance within Grace.

Travelling

Life is like a drive
In a slowly aging car.
There's much to see around us,
But focus where you are.

Intuition says, peer outward,
Keep the journey clear.
Strangely it's the opposite,
If you wish to hold what's dear.

Take care of your sleek auto,
It takes you everywhere.
But no matter how you care for it,
In time will disappear.

You are like a pilot,
That guides the auto on.
If fix your vision outward,
May never find your home.

So what's to say of journey
We're all pushed on to take?
The scenes of life go swiftly by,
Ever wonder at mistake?

Reflecting on the time that's past,
It seems that most do fine,
Until confronted with the fact
Their life is in decline.

Again it seems what's missing,
As we pilot selves along,
The needed pause to notice
Deep within we're not alone.

Behaviour has a consequence,
Some scoff at such a view.
But when your auto cease to be,
Who will you turn to?

The Spinning Wheel

The wheel is spinning faster,
With every passing day.
Appears it will not slow down
As it speeds us on our way.

Is it incidental, a bothersome effect?
Or can there be some meaning,
Of use,
To not neglect?

The problem is we think too much,
Our need to have control.
A comforting illusion,
So easy to extol.

Life is such a wonder,
But painful it can be.
There is struggle as we live it,
And a yearning to be free.

It's that yearning one might look at,
If can let go for a bit.
Recognise a whisper,
A sense mysterious.

Accept we know so little,
Fain to know so much!
Like bug in God's half acre,
We might be out of touch.

On internet are answers,
More than questions asked.
What is this life we're leading?
Reply, uneasy task.

Inward turn, a timeless place,
Will find no word to know.
Instead, a growing sense occurs,
A warming inner glow.

To Be Aware

Wonder at awareness?
The phenomenon itself?
Capacity to know you know,
Beyond at what is felt?

To explore the subtle nuance
Of what senses bring within.
To leave that realm, go deeper,
Where external seems to end.

To do so leaves awareness
Of a beauty that is you.
A calming sense of quiet,
Releasing, from the zoo.

To truly know the human being,
Not the brunt of something's joke.
The value you are held in,
Eternal's gentle stroke.

With patience and a gratitude,
What's found is wonder full.
Growing wisp of gentleness,
Sense Love beyond control.

To Be Authentic

To be authentic,
Can be a daunting task.
So important to be careful
Not to shake the other's mask.

Appear of interest, clever talk,
Keep it on the surface.
Stay away from personal,
Play it like a circus.

Because of such encounters,
They always take a toll,
A preference is for solitude,
To soothe a needy soul.

Away from all the chatter,
Aware of self, enhanced,
It soon becomes apparent,
How thinking sings and dance.

You begin to realise,
The mask is on you too.
We're all the same in depth, it seems,
But surface resists view.

Thinking creates clutter,
A constant, noisy buzz.
Fills the mind with fantasies,
Obscures what is beloved.

These fantasies, imaginings…
Can influence your choices,
From job career, to who you bed,
Like bewitching, siren voices.

It underscores ability
To find the empty space.
Where thought is gone, and what remains,
A sense of Loving Grace.

Cherished authenticity,
Has at last been gently found.
With end of all imaginings,
You find your Sacred Ground.

In the quiet, without thought,
Authentic you, ascends.
From this point, Reality,
Begins, and never ends.

The Wait

The fact that we're all simians
Is nothing one should flaunt.
It marks how low you wish to fall,
And that's a useless jaunt.

Sex, aggression, or display,
Can be fun, excite the mind,
But one thing we have little of,
Is precious, speeding time.

Youth burns fast, so use it well,
Don't waste it in the zoo.
There's more to us than thumping chest,
A consciousness, that's you.

Pause to wonder what's all this,
The bling, excitement's noise.
Try to balance carefully,
So not to lose your poise.

Find within a place to slow
The racing all around.
The point to your existence,
Is waiting to be found.

Mortal Roots

Not just descended from the ape,
We're close cousins, in our genes.
Offended by this simple fact?
Look closer at your dreams.

Check aggression.
Look at lust.
Throw in pride.
It's all of us.

Those offended put on airs,
Some will mock their brother.
It's kind of like a game we play,
Pathetic, hurt each other.

Without a clear acceptance
Of our roots in the primate,
Projection reigns, with attitude,
Leaving us prostrate.

Lack of self-awareness,
Numb to our inside,
Contributes rule of fantasy,
Desperate as we hide.

The goal is not for carnage,
To be feral and unkind.
Instead it is acceptance,
From there begin your climb.

A paradox is present,
In the helplessness one feels.
The less you sense yourself to be,
The closer to what's Real.

To recognise the primal,
But holding action firm,
One grows in self-awareness,
From there you slowly learn.

Cannot deny the ape,
Within we all do struggle.
But taming it needs consciousness,
Without which we are rubble.

So view your dogma holy,
As lift above another.
But listen to the whisper,
Of hubris, might then shudder.

Evil is a subtlety,
To watch with focal care.
Careful when belief leads you
To a privileged air.

Again, we all are primates,
No one, or group is more.
To entertain pretension,
A fantasy… deplore.

The genes dictate the animal.
Our consciousness ascends.
Place much into awareness,
To find it has no end.

Lift above the animal,
And trust in something more.
Discover with deep gratitude,
An inner Holy Door.

Moodiness

What is the swoon that takes us down,
Occurring for no clear reason?
And how is one to ascend again,
With thoughts that are heavy and weaken?

Life is dynamic,
With moods like the sea.
Swells of ascendance,
Descend frequently.

To be blessed with awareness
Enables to note,
It's thought to be helpless,
That grabs at the throat.

So thinking again,
Can cause our decline.
How does one deal
With such a design?

The hardware within
Is creature dependent.
The spirit it seems
Is always ascendant.

Reaching within,
Find humble demeanour.
Turning Above,
For support as believer.

Find a connection,
Through thankful reflection.
Uplifted, empowered,
A prized benediction.

Life's Mystery

Blessings, so profound to me,
Underscore the mystery.
So easy to be cavalier,
Assuming life is always clear.

Does control exist within our grasp?
Or only chance as time does pass?
Negating thoughts of strange events,
Assumed to be coincidence.

Puzzling it seems to be,
Alone is all that we can see.
If able to find time to pause,
Scan your life and look for cause.

Was blind luck the only take?
Or was there something having faith?
Unsettling are such thoughts to be,
A different view apparently.

It's been said in by gone days,
As things go well should be amazed.
When see of all that could go wrong
Life unfolds as if arranged.

Essentially just wish to say
Gratitude makes sense to feel.
We may be more than isolate,
Leaving wonder, what is real?

God's Will?

Sometimes I wonder,
What is God's Will?
Is it a reach?
Simply, vacuum to fill?

As event does unfold,
Such thoughts are in vain.
Posing such questions,
One is wilted and drained.

In tragedy's wake
Are empty discussions.
Serving no function,
Except for connections.

Again it appears,
Our fear of alone,
When stirred by disaster
We search for a Home.

It's almost as if
God's Will can be seen.
Relentless in urging,
A turn back to Him.

The move can be mocked
As foolish regression.
But it also can hint
At God's true intention.

Blaming

Blame, blame, blame.
Jung was right.
When terror strikes deep,
Make external strife.

Just pointing this out
As a thumb of rule.
When angst turns inward,
The outward turns cruel.

It's all quite simple,
All of us succumb.
Found in our genetics,
It's not that we are dumb.

So, when anger surges,
Social media perused,
Remember this as warning,
Angst can make us fools.

Aloneness

Aloneness we all struggle with,
It never goes away.
Diversions will be entertained,
In work as well as play.

What's the point to feel such pain?
The fear of dissolution?
How to fit the anguish viewed
In Darwin's evolution?

In due respect to science lore,
The animal its focus.
It might be best to look within,
Find numinous as locus.

Doing so will open up
A sense of grateful joy.
Aloneness is the animal.
Gentle fills the void.

Relating to the Infinite

Relation with the Infinite,
A view espoused by Tolstoy,
Defines what is religious,
Now troublesome to employ.

We scoff at such relations,
As illusory or worse,
Not recognising non-belief
As what may be perverse.

Religious need within us,
Manifests in many ways,
Instead of seeking Infinite,
With politics we play.

Entertain utopia,
Permitting all transgressions.
Be they sex, or all the same,
Excusing gross aggressions.

Chasing after empty fare,
Filled with childish yearning,
Talk of being comrades,
As sacred is left burning.

Instead of peering into self,
Where Infinity resides,
Projecting out from darkness
Our beast no longer hides.

A relation with the Infinite,
Is what we all are missing.
For morality and gentleness,
With finite in submission.

When pride is checked,
Our animal subdued,
The finite of our being
Brings Infinite in view.

As that which is eternal
Connects and resonates,
The sense of the religious
Is clear, and elevates.

Other

Have talked of the collective,
That group we all cling to;
Coercing one with subtlety,
Or ostracism cruel.

Frequently unnoticed,
Pressured to conform,
Generally ignored in life,
As long as uniform.

But when consciousness turns inward,
The group sees not at all,
Pressure then is brought to bear,
To deny what is recalled.

Is like the Inquisition,
Only now is much more subtle.
If try to hold collective's view,
The personal is muddled.

So, trust the self with inner strength,
A need to not be isolate.
Lean on what experienced,
The Other's strength inviolate.

Turning Attention

In our age of non-belief,
Where ideals appear quite trendy,
Searching through the ancient lore,
May seem a task too empty.

But finding time to turn a page,
Of what of old was honoured,
To read what's writ with patient mien,
Is rewarding to your ardour.

What offers much of such pursuit,
Is consciousness within us.
The musings of the older works,
Gives hints of what is timeless.

While set in different languages,
And culture influenced,
Thinking that is personal,
Informs, with proper prudence.

Sensing something more than us,
Pervades the sage abstractions.
Initially projecting out,
But then seen as reflections.

The frequency of such a view,
Gives interesting perspective.
Science works externally,
Results that are impressive!

But science struggles with what's in,
Finds difficult observing.
The expert, thus, of consciousness,
Is you and your enduring.

When note what ancients had to say,
Attention, turned in view.
More than just external fixed,
Turning, seeing you.

Allow yourself to settle in,
Recognise our debt.
Aware of something more than us,
A Presence beyond death.

The Question

The question rarely comes up,
As we coast along in life.
Seems we never pause to ask,
Until finding self in strife.

The question is a simple one,
No need to go to school.
Yet only when control is lost,
Does it cross the mind at all?

The question seems so basic,
But pursuit is rare to see.
Instead we turn to science,
To explain reality.

The question, from a primate,
It's what we really are,
Our pride tends to obscure that,
As evolution's scar.

The question still does linger,
May wonder why persists?
Is it Truth, or simple yearning,
To know God does exist?

The question isn't easy,
To find an answer to.
It remains a personal
Task for you to do.

The question doesn't fade away,
Unless defiance present.
Instead, a seeking inwardly,
May help you with its essence.

There's only one clear witness,
The experience is yours.
It's not a thought, or wishfulness,
But a strength that does endure.

The Meeting

Have often mulled life's mystery,
As toked a weed or two.
Dropping Acid was a trip,
Just once, as can undo.

Learning did occur with drugs,
But more clear when without.
Meaning did not clarify,
Was always left with doubt.

"Bonjour," she said, as left the cab,
Her sweetness was sincere.
Thus began our time of love,
And that was crystal clear.

When paused, to try and understand,
The thoughts led nowhere firm.
Experience what joy there was,
The only thing to learn.

As scanning all this life we lead,
Just live, is clear to be.
But having thought capacity
Can lead to misery.

Thinking yields a field of doubt,
From there to pain and loss.
So joy of love soon dissipates,
Appears thought has its cost.

Parting, left in grief alone,
A lesson terribly learned.
It's not the thought, to analyse,
But growth of love, not spurned.

Yearning for her sweet embrace,
Open to the wonder.
Thinking put aside from us,
Doubt is torn asunder.

Returning to the both of us,
The point of life more clear.
It's hope and fullness through embrace,
And sense of love held dear.

Subjectivity

A sweet word, such as obfuscate,
Is clearly on the mark,
As struggle with our thinking,
And theological thought.

Experience subjective,
With comprehensive haze.
Even Paul, Damascus bound,
Heaven sense, is vague.

The human need for order,
Transcends what can be sensed.
Confabulation frequent,
When faced with ignorance.

Not negating spirit,
Or Holy words received.
Simply pointing out,
Why there are so many creeds.

Experience is valid,
Translation may be poor.
Evidence for Mystery
Can shrink to mere folklore.

What's the point of seeking,
If thought can lead astray?
It's the personal experience,
Like Love felt, as you pray.

Primate Residue

There is a view of evil,
And many others too,
That says that it exists in us,
As primate residue.

And only if we see it,
Accept as part of us,
Will it be caged and reined in?
From there we can adjust.

But if this evil, in us,
Is denied or spread about,
It gathers strength dispersing,
No difference what its route.

We try to think of reasons,
For it creeping everywhere.
But find our logic feeble,
Thus left with dark despair.

Only when we recognise,
The evil in ourselves,
Can control be in the grasp,
And darkness be dispelled.

The tragic truth of history is
Such a goal elusive?
We tend to think collectively,
Not singular exclusive.

Perhaps a frequent pause to peer,
A moment to reflect.
To look within the heart of us,
Our self to not neglect.

Such effort seems more relevant,
As community entwine.
To underscore one's specialness,
And find what does malign.

This viewpoint may be difficult,
Accepting us, as is.
But remember Doctor Jekyll?
His story reflects this.

To power over others,
Being in control.
Reaching out material,
Coerce to gain a goal.

These and many others,
Clear demonic fodder.
Thus reaching inward to the self,
To illuminate and collar.

Power of Thought

The power of thought
Can be quite devastating.
Conception, imagining,
Corrupt, elevating.

A fantasy spun,
Regarding another.
When fractured by real,
Can tear self-asunder.

Imagining romance,
Finding not so.
Feeling abashed,
Control is let go.

More fantasy spin,
Like grasping for straw.
Thoughts without number,
As balance is sought.

The disruption that's noted,
Causing distress,
Is connection that's lost,
Sense free-fall at best.

Connection essential,
Our beast needs its hold.
Without firm connecting,
Terror unfolds.

Some have awareness,
As body parts fail.
Others stay panicked,
But hide as they flail.

When find quiet moments,
With thought that's subdued,
A peace can be seen,
Will find more of you.

As thinking is muted,
With calming that's found,
A hold that is gentle,
Is felt as profound.

Comfort observed,
Gratitude clear,
Perhaps prayer expressed,
To Something that's near.

Whatever is felt,
As peace is perceived,
Connection occurs,
To Something received.

No explanation
Is easily found,
Left feeling grateful,
For Ultimate Ground.

Our Unconscious

It's believed by some
That God is within,
And out,
An archetype of sorts.

Found in dreams,
Or deep in prayer,
That is,
What they report.

It's said that He exists,
In the unconscious of us all.
That we have a task to reach within,
To hopefully recall.

If neglect, or leave untouched,
Reach not to sense His presence,
Danger then presents to us,
Mistake our ego, for His Essence.

The hubris that mars our time,
With boundaries vague, or gone,
Conviction we create ourselves,
Control earth's weather song.

Looking up to science,
As the saviour we all seek.
Needing to turn inward,
An effort all too weak.

Finding we're hard-wired,
Perceiving in, as out.
It's easy to have lassitude,
At best to simply doubt.

This is offered as reflection
That some have, of what's within,
A fascinating viewpoint,
As seek a sense of Him.

Guilt – Some Thoughts

Been thinking of guilt, ubiquitous,
The pain is very sad.
It's even with the psychopath,
But deep below a slab.

The use in Social Contract,
Too obvious to state.
It thrives in all our fantasies,
Haunts and creates ache.

Useful to keep order,
Not operate alone.
Can cause distorted thinking,
Disrupt a peaceful home.

Try to rid ourselves of it,
Project and point to other.
Never really works too well,
Tears everyone asunder.

How to ease the pain?
Be free without regret?
Perhaps to understand a key…
It's aloneness, disconnect.

Some may say that's nonsense,
With energy may scoff.
But if they pause a little bit,
Find ardour covers rot.

Relief occurs when shared with other,
Only for a while.
A chronic sense of guilt persists,
That wipes away a smile.

Strangely it is found,
When pause a bit, reflect.
That turning in and upward,
With supplicated wit…

A calming can be noted,
But reason stays unclear.
As pray to find forgiveness,
With reach to have One near.

If it is connection,
That offers peace at last,
Seems Ultimate Relationship,
Can never be surpassed.

On Birthdays

A thought to share, this sacred time,
The memory of your birth.
So easy seems, to blow it off,
As simply time for mirth.

The fact remains it marks a pause,
When nothing seemed to matter.
Nothing but the cry you sobbed,
As consciousness was gathered.

So easy it does seem to be
To take all life on surface.
The breath you took began a trip,
Like running through a circus.

But should you pause to catch your breath,
And peer in you, a bit,
It might be found there's more to you
Than simple old habit.

To know, you know, amazing!
And a wonder to behold!
The consciousness you truly are,
Timeless and quite old.

So have a sweet, good birth day,
Remember who you are.
Not a creature grasping,
But a conscious soul and star.

On Anger

Anger is like oil spill,
Where control has oozed away.
It stains all that is close to it,
Intention not in play.

Once that it is triggered
It permeates your scene.
Whatever hope for caring,
Is gone, no more serene.

The Dove you closely treasured,
Is covered in the goo.
Rage that's deep inside,
Has taken over you.

Like spills it cleans up slowly,
No matter how you try.
It's best to pull away from all,
Perhaps to even cry.

An irony that must be shared,
Is the driving force of rage.
It's deeper guilt, perhaps not felt,
That burns at every stage.

Guilt hints at loss, oblivion,
To end up all alone.
Self-punishing, the impulse is,
Fearing loss of home.

What's the answer for such ire,
How regain control?
Feel forgiven quells the fire,
Find what's very Old.

Journey

Of interest it may be,
Without hyperbole,
The measure of one's self,
Is not in books on shelf.

Nor in texts of social norms,
In science or statistics.
A fact remains, each lives inside,
We are our own true critics.

Many don't peer in that much,
Fixed on outward signs.
Leaving shells of human beings,
Not seen, except their rinds.

Such mortals waste their time,
Given as a gift.
Pursuing the material,
Soul cut loose to drift.

But if attend, with quiet mien,
To what resides within,
There's found the truth about one's self,
It's where your task begins.

To know your truth is painful,
We're not what hoped to be.
The limit, that is found of us,
Gives help to clearly see.

The smaller you experience,
And errors you have made,
A sense of guilt and evil,
Leaves despair a growing wave.

But patience, with a touch of faith,
Will help you to recover,
The soul that is within you,
With gentleness uncover.

Growing in awareness,
Of what is more than life,
Despair gives way to gratitude,
And gloom gives way to light.

Islands

Ever feel apologetic
Simply to exist?
Never really fitting in,
Apart from all the rest.

Others seem accepted
In groups they hang around.
But if you peer more closely,
Something similar is found.

It's the island we all are,
As we spot the sea we're in.
Reaching for connection,
Afraid to dive and swim.

At times there is a union,
Two islands flow and touch.
But still there is a separateness,
That leaves one not so much.

The sea is like the numinous,
Surrounds us everywhere.
But as we are like islands,
It leaves us in despair.

We desire for connecting,
A sense to unify.
But in our self-absorption,
Seems easy to get by.

The planet that we drift on
Is whole and holds us all.
But lacking in perspective,
It's fragments we recall.

On our little islands,
Fantasy does fly.
Each creates an idol,
That is worshipped 'til we die.

The unity that's present,
Is missed by most it seems.
They just keep on drifting,
Left with hopeless dreams.

To obtain a right perspective,
Take in, all that you are.
Note that something holds you,
No matter near or far.

The island that you thought you were,
Dissolves into the sea.
Yet you remain a clarity,
Beyond what used to be.

Inward Side

I'm amazed at simplicity
Of all that we see,
When in fact it reflects
A deep mystery,

Looking about a simple room,
Nothing very special,
When thoughts on hold, it changes some,
Almost reverential.

Reflect, is a fine word,
To describe what's all around,
As we receive the images,
Of sight, and touch, and sound.

The data that we process,
Is chemically transformed,
Our consciousness observes this,
Puts us out there since we're born.

We tend to lose sight
Of the inner world of us,
Occupied with busyness,
There's loss of inner trust.

The loss is quite profound, it seems,
For within is found what's Real,
It's not illusion, stuff of dreams,
More than what you feel.

Experience is personal,
A point to underscore,
It's easy to forget ourselves,
A fact we should deplore.

Attention to the inward side,
Of what we see out there,
Can bring us closer to what's Real,
Increase our sense of care.

When thought desist, the self pursued,
Wonder does expand,
A sense of growing gratitude,
As gentle as a lamb.

Direction

Ever notice when upset
Thoughts act as little logs.
Thrown in the fire's rage,
They help flame it along.

Try you may, they can't be stopped,
Heat keeps on rising up.
And under it, attend if can,
An angst produces thought.

Find the angst, if can discover,
The heat begins to wane.
Feel a sense of some discomfort,
In the belly there is pain.

The angst is terror, undefined,
The beast within is loose.
Creature, try so hard to hide,
Is shaking off its noose.

It uses what we pride to have,
Our thinking as a tool.
Instead of creativity,
It rages like a bull.

So here's a plan that might be used,
To settle down the angst.
Turn to spirit, connection sought,
In quiet, offer thanks.

Depth of Life

There's more to this life,
Than appears at a glance.
Much that occurs
Is not just by chance.

We stay on its surface
Don't pause to look in.
Missing the point,
Our vision stays dim.

Easy to miss
A pattern that's there.
Accepting as luck
What may reflect care.

Focus on work,
Moments of fun.
What seems without meaning,
May not be humdrum.

With no inward peering,
Life seems simple and clear.
The problem, however,
No meaning appears.

But, may not be pointless,
Empty and harsh.
You may have a soul,
Take care it's not lost.

When begin to suspect
A Hand that's not seen.
There's growth in thanks giving,
As Love fills your being.

Counting Blessings

When one comes up empty,
On contemplative fare.
Feeling all futility.
That nothing's really there.

Add the sense of meaningless,
Or worse, a pang of guilt,
Stirring shades of darkness,
Surrounded by a pelt.

The poverty of hopefulness,
Too painful to endure,
Can lead you to the seeking
For something clean and pure.

At such hopeless moments,
In silent reverie,
Turn attention fully
To gifts you have received.

Find what is a blessing,
That you exist at all.
Begin to wonder gently,
Is there something to recall?

The mystery of being,
Persists throughout one's life.
Events shrugged off as accident,
May reflect His Light.

With patience can be found
A sense of Presence dear.
The counting of one's blessings,
Can bring this very near.

There are no thoughts expressing such,
It's feeling and a sense.
Know clearly in the mind
A Truth in its essence.

Illusion or delusion?
A call for those 'who know'?
But if your vision's inward,
You're really on your own.

Confusion

Were we to live one thousand years,
A life of questioned value.
It's said the rich transfuse with youth;
Take care of what they sell you.

The search goes on, will never end,
For youthful raw elixir.
To find a way, no matter how,
To slow our ailing mixture.

In past pursued by Alchemy,
The sacred Holy Grail.
Confusing spirit, blessed
For raw material.

This confusion clearly moves
The wealthy and much more.
Perhaps they'll find what's sought so dear,
Results they may deplore.

The error seems ubiquitous,
With those appearing smart.
They follow cold material,
Instead of in their heart.

It's grasping and controlling
That stirs the growth of greed.
Instead of peering inward,
Aware of their true need.

Raises constant questions
Of what is life about?
To lift above the animal?
Appears a humble start.

But in these times of hubris,
Where we create ourselves,
To look within is mocked, or rare,
Awareness left on shelves.

We idolise our brethren,
Forgetting, they're no more than you.
Constant reaching for a star,
A fixed external view.

In prayer or meditation
Can seek what is within,
But notice the aversion
Our culture leaves us in?

Discomfort with the numinous,
As if it would be weird,
To be a gentle seeker,
Who's looking for His Word.

All this is to share,
A simple point of view,
There's need for inward peering,
To find what's truly you.

Cautious Progress

Science has progressed it seems,
Beyond our expectations.
In medicine and other fields,
Appears no limitations.

Able to turn gender
Any way it wants.
Yielding fine results at ease,
Amusing as it jaunts.

There appears no limit,
In direction it can take.
The body remains malleable,
Seems easy to create.

There's a creature at our root,
Permeates all we do.
The more we try to hide it,
The more it filters through.

With power that seems limitless,
The primate stirs its claws.
It scratches to pursue a task
As if there were no Laws.

What's missing in the scientist,
And others of us too,
Value of the human being…
Not evolution's view.

More than just organic.
Possessing soul that lifts.
A counter to the animal,
The reason we exist?

With values that are vague,
Ideals diversified,
Without a sense of Deity,
The brute in us can thrive.

Maybe this exaggerates
A danger to beware.
But watch extremes of medicine,
Note creature lurking there.

Borrowed Time

We're all on borrowed time,
But the debt is not observed.
It's wasted on frivolity,
No wish to be unnerved.

The gift of self-awareness,
So precious and pristine,
Exploited or neglected,
To maintain one's self-esteem.

A pause, that's so important,
To look within one's self,
So easy to neglect,
As we run in search of wealth.

The time we have, a gift,
Would seem that's very clear.
Might open up our consciousness.
To thankfulness sincere.

Instead we stay on surface,
Take life as it glides by.
Work and play, take in a show,
Might comment, "Time does fly!"

Again, the question may arise,
What point is all the fuss?
An answer seems a beckoning,
As true for all of us.

It's love that is another gift,
A measure of our reach.
When young can be capricious,
In time has much to teach.

Were we to pause and wonder,
Suspect there's more than seen.
Might come to slowly realise,
The soul within our being.

Blessings?

It's hard to write on blessings,
In this culture we're all in.
Too easy to be viewed,
As naive and maybe dim.

Yet looking at our lives,
As travel through all time,
It's difficult to view as luck,
What's good and so sublime.

The awful things that happen
To innocence is real.
No way to figure reason,
Or justify what's ill.

Thinking is obscuring,
Arrogance is worse.
Viewing all material,
Existence made a curse.

When heads rolled into baskets,
Some would crow with glee,
Bringing down the privileged,
Including royalty.

While cleansing much corruption,
Ridding empty fools,
It never did occur to them,
They're cutting off our souls.

Terror stifles spirit,
Stirs the creature's bed,
Leads away from good intent,
To arrogance and dread.

Remains of countries ravaged,
The terror/rage is spent.
A growing sense of emptiness,
An existential rent.

Medieval reaching upward,
Now a horizontal grasp.
Material ascendent,
Spirit viewed as past.

Ideals have fallen downward,
A collective view and quest.
Our creation lost in hubris,
The creature knows what's best.

Yet single is the power,
To balance and recover.
Finding as peer inward,
A whisper sense of Other.

A sense that is a Mystery
If pause and look within.
Negates the seeming emptiness,
In world of flesh and din.

Chasing Ideals

You can engineer a rocket,
You can engineer a tool,
But engineering people,
Can only lead to cruel.

Anarchists will tear down,
To build their ideal state,
Not smart enough to realise,
Ideals deteriorate.

Idealistic communes,
Are exactly that.
Reality is limiting,
Simply read the facts.

In the nineteenth century,
Many communes were designed.
Utopias in hopefulness,
But everyone declined.

All communistic systems,
Have failed through history.
Initially ideal,
Then coercive of the free.

It seems that ideal systems,
Work best for the designer.
They decline as spin to others,
Free will is the definer.

So careful as you search
For ideals, to make them real.
Ideals are what we reach for,
But grasping is futile.

There is religious principle,
Within it does reside.
It reflects what is Ideal,
As the ultimate of High.

This is not the secular,
But religious hope of future.
The turn should be to inward growth,
A sacred quest adventure.

You can engineer a rocket,
You can engineer a tool,
But engineering people
Will result in loss of soul.

Always Questions

If God is within,
And also out,
Appears it is known,
What we're all about.

If such not true,
And thus all alone,
Would seem we are free,
Simply to roam.

But guilt and shame,
Persist in most,
As if we all,
Exist as host.

Simply learned?
A sense of care?
Or is there something
Put it there?

Then there's that religious sense,
Many have experienced.
It lightens up one's inner being,
With Love, it's light, and sense of freeing.

More is in, than we can know,
May lead us to an inner glow.
Comfort found within its fold,
Perhaps to sense a gentle hold.

Leaving one with gratitude,
Feeling Care and Love.
Experience humility,
And wonder at Above.

A Puzzle

Isn't it odd,
How we struggle to begin?
To know that life's reflected,
When attention is turned in?

Plato said it clearly,
In his story of the Cave.
That all that's known are shadows,
From which ideas are made.

We don't appear hung up,
That our inner self is vague.
Instead is chased material,
Absorbed in primal clay.

Our consciousness, so special,
Has served us wonderfully.
But fixed on the external,
There's Truth that is not seen.

Hidden, but decisive,
Is the primate that we are.
Pushing out to action,
From self to move afar.

If only one could pause a bit,
To look within, and hone;
Over-ride the animal,
Find we're not alone.

The flesh, that is our vehicle,
Made creature over time.
Evolved to master all around,
The self, it does deny.

Woe to us, absorbed as such,
Not noting that we're foolish.
AI created masterly,
Smart but dreadful soulless.

As noted, it seems odd,
The struggle that exists.
For each and every one of us,
To not search within for bliss.

Home

Jung said it best,
So many years ago.
It is not what's believed,
It's really what you know.

Thought is always useful,
But it also can deceive.
Trust in your experience,
Greater clarity received.

Now, maybe you're deluded,
In illusion, something more.
But it also may be solid,
A Reality to adore.

Trust yourself a bit,
Resist collective pressure.
Hold to what's experienced,
Your self to be the measure.

This life is very short,
Much to be accomplished.
Put more will into the self,
To find what is your true wish.

Others may disparage,
As if they alone are clear.
Recognise what's personal,
Only you can find what's dear.

As become more focused,
To a hold, that is a Singular,
In collective, lost you were,
You now see more particular.

It's amazing to achieve this,
To stand, yourself, alone.
But finding this ability,
Brings you back to Home.

Celebrity

The problem being human,
Is the animal we are.
One can be an icon,
Perhaps a movie star.

Believing all the media,
Comfort with your skills.
Finding you have influence,
The ego overfills.

Of all the flaws found present,
Be they sex, or greed, or drugs.
The one that eats away with pride,
Is mortal sting, with no Above.

As long as flow with power swift,
Blind to passing time.
Caught up in self-inflated drift,
Illusion does entwine.

Religious sense, that drives ideals,
Scattered in false climbs.
As mortal grows in certitude,
Imbalance is the sign.

Secretly the angst does grow,
No comment to your fans.
Alone in darkness turn to know,
A dread that does expand.

"Why this dread?", the thought occurs,
Unclear, despair fills in.
Religious sense, that's been ignored,
A secret, quiet Friend.

You see, it's lost connection,
That the animal despairs.
The primate that we all are,
Sees only earthly cares.

There is a sense of spirit,
That needs you to attend.
Let go your pride-filled stubbornness,
To find you're without end.

Choice

We see breadth of reality,
But take too much for granted.
Assure ourselves of what is real,
To not be disenchanted.

It seems we are suggestible,
Through our education.
Whether family, school, or media,
We're locked in soft persuasion.

This creates an attitude,
Preconception flourishing.
Material our chosen view,
All else is seen discouraging.

It is a pity, it's a shame,
Our view is kept so narrow.
A Reality so filled with joy,
Instead chose empty barrow.

Acceleration

Science is but few years old,
A breath or maybe six.
Civilisation several thousand,
Not much when you reflect.

Gods have brought us much our way,
Revered and sought for guidance.
Our sacred view held preciously,
To it we turned in silence.

But swiftly started questioning,
Darwin fed the view,
Maybe gods are simply us,
Created, then we slew.

Even sense of God has grown,
Over last few thousand years.
But slaying our divinity,
Seems how we deal with fear.

Finding us much more alone,
No divinity to turn to,
Religious sense made politic,
Heaven on Earth the new view.

Still remains a question,
For us creatures newly formed.
Why the sense of sacredness,
If all alone we're born?

Seems an odd experience,
To feel there's so much more.
We blow it off as wanderlust,
When it may be sacred's call.

So hesitant we seem to be,
To reach in, for what is numinous.
As if to fear what's more than us,
Chose darkness, not the luminous.

So here we are, alone with tools,
Creating us in frenzy.
Leaving secret, aloneness fear,
Our pride acts as a sentry.

Maybe God has not been slain,
But calls to us to listen.
Leaving each with will to choose,
To find we've all been christened.

Guilt – An Introduction

Let go the mystic,
And turn to the mental.
Guilt pervades us,
It's elemental.

Freud called it,
The superego.
Name what you like,
It haunts all us people.

The irony and power,
It tends to present,
At first glance is good,
But in depth decadent.

Can feed mindless rage,
Or cause self-destruction.
Helps with relations,
But freedom reduction.

It's the thinking inside,
The whispers deceitful,
That torture and chide,
Leaving you grief full.

Alone with the struggle,
Difficult task.
Battle with guilt,
A thought-filled morass.

At some point turn upward,
Look for forgiveness.
Find comfort in Love,
Its essence, mysterious.

Wonderland

There always is a mystery
In this wonder-filled voyage.
It's the irony we live in,
What's real or just mirage.

Like Alice in her Wonderland,
Wide eyed, we take it in.
Behind the scenes presented us,
Queen of Hearts will cause our end.

There is no rhyme or reason,
For her constant hatefulness.
She's ruler of the kingdom,
To her, He has forsaken us.

So on we go,
Taking as presented.
A party with some tea cups,
Feeling discontented.

Madness all around us,
Seeking a way out.
How to find the rabbit hole?
Up rise, and turnabout.

Perhaps that is a narrow view,
Fed by all unhinged.
It's not a hidden passageway,
But where it's always been.

Every one of us,
Is secretly immortal.
Because there's so much noise and fuss,
Out soul becomes too subtle.

Pause a bit, and turn within,
Look to what is Real.
Find what's not forsaken us.
Through Love, you find the Seal.

Inner Strength

We have this heightened consciousness,
And sharpened tool of thought.
There's no more fur to burden us,
We're upright as we walk.

Much of our appearance,
Seems less of being feral.
Can fool ourselves believing,
We're godlike, to our peril.

This sense is fed by markets,
Selling meat in tidy package.
Leaving the impression,
No animal's been savaged.

Much of how we do life,
With tools that dazzle mind,
Offers us impression,
That we are indeed divine.

Alas, when something happens,
Unplanned and overwhelming.
Leaves us feeling smaller,
Our weakness quite compelling.

Events like these are useful,
They help us hearken back,
To time we roamed the tundra,
Reached up for what we lacked.

The point is it is helplessness,
That urges turning in.
To recognise our rootedness,
As creatures in the end.

Leave divine to what's beyond,
Our feeble comprehension.
Not foolish in our self to be,
Accede to apprehension.

Knowing just how small we are,
The universe quite massive.
Allow yourself to turn a glance,
To something sheer impressive.

More than us, with all we are,
A comfort when adrift.
Sensing frail enfeeblement,
But strengthened by His Grip.

Connection Within

It's tough when one suspects a Truth,
In this culture we reside.
Having folk with outer view,
Believe they can deride.

Facts they have, consensus drawn,
Collective they are strong.
Never really thinking clear,
As group they may be wrong.

Grouping is the strongest point,
That nature can provide.
At least this true for primates,
For eons kept alive.

But with ascent of consciousness,
Free will does intervene.
Accentuating singular,
Each searching for a meaning.

So easy to accommodate,
To outer points of view,
To lose our singularity,
As one, is very few.

Within one's self are darkened fears,
The collective can assuage.
Less lonely in collective's fold,
Believe in mindless fate.

Yet each exist within one's self,
With joy, despair, and hope,
Each seeking satisfaction,
In a life that's hard to cope.

The key to understanding,
To peer inward more than out,
Is recognise connection,
As what we're all about.

Finding a relationship,
Imbued with Loving care,
Offers individual,
A counter to despair.

Copernicus

Copernicus moved us from the centre,
The earth around the sun.
It seems the same for consciousness,
Within were not sovran.

Difficult to accept this,
Especially when young.
But as we move along in years,
No longer number one.

To achieve this view with clarity,
Hubris needs to shrink.
The sense of all important,
An illusion as you think.

Much of life illusory,
As thought spins out its web.
Keeping all preoccupied,
Leaving us mislead.

Material quite seductive,
With pleasure and its glitter.
Spirit sense neglected,
Empty and embittered.

Years drift by like paper shreds.
Meaning slips away.
Continued self-importance,
Empty in its wake.

But as grow in self-awareness,
Suspect one not alone,
Finding greater consciousness,
Above what was called home.

Feeling small and helpless,
But growing clear and pure.
Turn to Love's enlightenment,
His consciousness secured.

Imitation

Connection and identify,
Reflect an imitation.
This is what the monkey does,
Since early in creation.

Our self is lost in multitude,
This without intention.
Each one of us gives up unique,
Conscious in suspension.

There's chasing after money,
Prestige, and power too,
All reaching out to nothingness,
But illusion is our school.

Because the I is fixed on other,
Confusion who we are.
Rage or triumph with them all,
Our self seen from afar.

This will tend to go unnoticed,
Throughout one's early years.
Jung suggests about midlife,
Questions may appear.

Reflecting on one's life gone by,
With inward turn of gaze.
The monkey that we struggle with,
Is seen through thought-filled haze.

Once viewed as ape, we really are,
With vision inward focused,
Control comes through our consciousness,
We then know our true locus.

No need denial, projection checked,
Our task is deeply closet.
Forgiveness sought, wrongs more clear,
Humility upon us.

As you single, self alone,
Silence is oppressive.
But then a subtle warmth appears,
It's Love that is connective.

Inclusive

The essence of evil,
Is descent to emptiness.
Accompanied by sensory,
Agitated fest.

Drugs are very useful,
Attaining such a state.
Heighten sense of consciousness,
Where carnal dominates.

Appear to reach the animal,
With zoologic zeal.
Feeling superhuman,
A kind of god appeal.

Illusion that is inward,
Instead of outward strewn.
How fantasy appeals to us,
What's real has little room.

Left with clear frustration,
With what is poor in time.
Searching for Reality,
Diverted from sublime.

Each of us important,
As we stand alone beseeching.
Praying for responsiveness,
From silence we keep reaching.

Strange and yet so wonderful,
You don't remain evasive.
Find that inward quietness,
Forgiveness grows pervasive.

At such moments held so dear,
It becomes more lucid.
That You are simply very clear,
It's Love that is inclusive.

Feeling

God's image appears,
To vary with thought.
Each person a view,
Can be subtle, or not.

Seems as we try,
Put into words,
Our nature entwines,
Create what we yearn.

This can suggest,
We worship a dream,
Something of us,
That we make supreme.

All this to say,
Take care what you think.
Still, the sense of Above,
May not be extinct.

The value of thought,
Absurd to neglect,
We're more than cognition,
Not to forget.

Even belief,
Is thought in itself,
Can be debated,
Differs from felt.

Thus conviction resides,
In you, and your senses.
Acceptance is yours,
Try not to build fences.

Thinking a tool,
A wonder to have,
But can cause distraction,
The loss would be sad.

Busy with doubt,
And endless debating.
Missing what's felt,
Promoting its fading.

The Truth can be found,
Residing in you.
If pause between thought,
To find a new view.

What's felt is a scene,
For you as partaker.
It's yours to receive,
Between you and your Maker.

Inner View

Here's another thought,
For those not so inclined.
Maybe would be helpful,
To open up the mind.

It seems if pause to notice,
The self in world surround,
Attend to quiet breathing,
As the only chafing sound.

Awareness of this inner view,
Of all the outside scene,
Slowly 'comes apparent,
Of what you might be seeing.

This becomes important,
For growth in clarity.
It emphasises consciousness,
Within disparity.

It's the consciousness of self,
That would be emphasised.
This begins awareness,
It opens up your eyes.

So doing, yields a feeling,
Of excitement and of hope.
Achieving new perspective,
A different way to cope.

Perhaps it is the emphasis,
On self that does occur.
Attending more to you at last,
Conformity discouraged.

Awareness of the inner world,
Coexisting with the other.
A greater sense of numinous,
No longer undercover.

However you define it,
Whatever view is stressed,
When underscore the sense of you,
Centrality is best.

Not a note of arrogance,
Nor foolish self-indulgence,
But seeing life as truly is,
Achieving clear intelligence.

A point that is important,
Too much of the above,
Is from the self, to world,
Opens you to Love.

Mind

Reviewing many writers,
Jung is a good read,
Finding that what works for them,
May not work for me.

This does not disparage,
Their thoughts, so fine and clear.
It only is to underscore,
That personal is dear.

If you're not the expert,
On what inside you find,
Then illusion is the irony,
As originates outside.

It's easy to forget,
The self that is in you.
To intoxicate the mind,
Absorbed with different view.

So when unclear, the point of what is all,
Get tips from what is read.
But the source you might be searching for
Is really in your head.

Pathway

To look at life spread out before us,
In space or simply time,
It's never smooth or easy going,
Not what one would call sublime.

The journey's tough, yet captivating,
In many ways a challenge.
It yields rewards, and specialness,
Can leave one feeling boundless.

But as it's lived with hope and joy,
If pause and life reflect,
May find a quiet restlessness,
As if some self-neglect.

When years pass, with much achieved,
Begin to wonder why?
The animal is satisfied,
But something in you chides.

It's strange that it is difficult
To find one's sense of self.
That quality, so personal,
Deep within what's felt.

Perhaps we're all so dizzy
With our animal pursuits,
We cannot turn attention,
To what grows above our roots.

You have to peer within yourself,
Reach up instead of down.
Let go the need for rational,
Accept what is profound.

Clearly thought is priceless,
Understanding is its essence,
But intuition, inner sight,
Can lead you to a Presence.

Presence

I find when live without a spirit sense,
Alone but filled with joy.
Occupied with stirring fare,
To keep one's mind employed.

That questions existential,
Are very far away.
Such interests do not bother one,
To them you do not stray.

But slowing down, control not clear,
Perspective seems to shift.
Uneasiness appears to stir,
The mind feels cut adrift.

Perhaps the mortal that we are,
No longer is denied,
The sense of growing nothingness,
More difficult to hide.

Some view this, as all there is,
The spirit weak to see.
That science will solve everything,
The rest is fantasy.

Perhaps this view has merit,
Perhaps it's credible,
But personal experience,
Reveals exceptional.

When settle in, to one self-true,
The noise outside abated,
It's found a glow of something more,
Aloneness is negated.

As trust this sense, allow to be,
Know grateful and revere.
Feel a loving warmth to grow,
A Presence ever near.

River's Course

Life is like a river.
Without a reason why.
We drift into swift currents,
That throw us as we ride,

There is no explanation,
Of why such wrath occurs,
It's the nature of the river,
The course can't be deterred.

But as we travel on it,
Take note of how it churns,
Soon after rapids settle,
A calm and beauty stirs.

So find within acceptance,
There's no control to have.
Be thankful for the journey,
For consciousness, be glad.

Simplicity

Some turn to the East,
Some to the West.
Who is to know,
Which direction is best?

The human of us,
Thinks we are quite smart.
Care should be present
As find guru to start.

It appears, if are honest,
Decision is yours,
A choice of a mentor,
Is exterior.

Might ponder to find,
A direction to choose.
A turn to peer inward,
Find expert is you!

Solace

There are those profess to know,
Emerson called it Over-Soul.
I have often said it clear,
I do not know, but still revere.

To have a sense of something more,
Not belief, a different door.
Experience without a thought,
Finding what is simply sought.

Not hallucination strong,
Nor illusions to enthral.
Instead a hint of mystery,
With no thought of sophistry.

Enraptured by the touch of Love,
And gratitude to what's above.
Review of life's events and such,
Having Grace, we owe so much.

Many find this not enough,
Wanting proof, or heady stuff.
As if this precious life of ours,
Did not excite like games for hours.

Seems there is a comforting,
When rest within the self.
Not for proof or lecturing,
The solace is enough.

Gift or Chance?

Sometimes I just fill up,
With thankfulness and bliss.
To know a simple fact as such;
That is, that I exist.

The capacity to self-reflect,
Learn values and much more.
To know that there's a universe,
Just waiting to explore.

A sense of endless mystery,
We try in vain to answer.
Our fancy running wild, unleashed,
Like a dizzy dancer.

The wonder isn't just out there,
It also lies within.
There is so much that is unclear,
Our knowledge remains thin.

A thought exists that earth itself,
Is consciousness we are.
Like cells that make the brain of us,
We make the mind of Terra.

Such thoughts lead one to blind conviction,
That, to mass enthralled.
Singular becomes diminished,
Lost to Siren's call.

Seems the individual,
Has need to be with other.
To recognise aloneness,
Stirs fright of blown asunder.

What if conscious sense of us,
Is not just evolved chance?
Instead it be a blessedness,
To find the self-enhanced.

A blessing hints at Giver,
Something more than us.
It takes away the loneliness,
Leaves you more than dust.

However, you may view it,
A gift, or merely chance,
To know you are a knower,
One becomes enhanced.

Recognise it as a boon,
Leaves humility, delight.
Aware of something Sacred,
Comfort throughout life.

The Navigator

We are much of what we download,
A lot is brought in too.
Hiding what is deep within,
We're kind of like a zoo.

All of evolution,
Resides within our depth.
Free will is on the surface,
There's power below deck.

Sailing to adventure,
Routine is common place.
Touching in on countless ports,
Enriched by interface.

Navigation helps to guide,
Direct one's course of action.
Some ignore the stars above,
No purpose, just distraction.

We live in times of disbelief,
Depend on one another.
Navigate by turn to stars?
Viewed foolish and a bother.

So on your deck are views and thought,
Their numbers keep on climbing.
Wandering the sea with doubt,
Feel lost, no goal worth finding.

There's darkness in the boat we are,
Unexplored, and frightening.
Our animal is powerful,
Constantly inciting.

We fool ourselves with intellect,
To hide what's really feral.
Unless it's seen within ourselves,
Projects outside as terrible.

The Navigator that we need,
Is clever and perceptive.
He sees each launch within itself,
To help us find perspective.

Thus importance of a Guide,
To reach above the din.
Sail ourselves, clear goal in mind,
Not lost when we have Him.

The Shelf

As we age, the body does,
At times can be discouraging.
If quite clear, know where to look,
Can find what is encouraging.

Our consciousness appears to be,
The central sense of self.
But if attend more carefully,
Will find it's just a shelf.

Below the shelf are secrets,
Above it more than you.
Appears there is awareness,
All around our simple view.

Difficult accepting
We're not the number one.
But when aware of smallness,
Our vanity's undone.

Like we did discover,
That earth circles the sun,
It's also true of ego,
Around Almighty's One.

So when there is unhappiness,
Or fear of cancellation,
Turn attention to within,
Discover supplication.

To know our small enfeeblement,
But not be fear possessed.
Recognise Another's Grace,
Within, His hold to rest.

Ubiquitous Primate

You can put a rose, on an animal's ear,
Or blanket with bouquet.
It still remains an animal,
In spite of overlay.

So it is with culture,
Promoted by our thought.
Appearance it does underscore,
Hiding what's corrupt.

Jung emphasised the shadow,
Freud put forth the id.
Whatever one may call it,
Evil remains hid.

Easy to psychologise,
As grapple with this blot.
Mental acrobatics,
To insist what one is not.

When projection is found useful,
To be rid of one's disgust.
What might have been self-loathing,
Is turned to other's rut.

Without a patient reading,
Of what resides within,
We continue to look outwards,
Blaming folk for our own sin.

Thus, this is to emphasise,
The need for inward peering.
Doing so gives conscious light,
To what you had been fearing.

The answer to the primate,
That is struggled deep within,
Is something that is more than us,
A reach beyond our kin.

Seems when move to silence,
Between each thought we have,
Feel less self-important,
Our claws begin to flag.

No reason seems apparent,
For why this does occur.
Other than beyond our wit,
A Presence does endure.

Waiting

I must admit to waiting,
With a quiet reverie.
Trying not to think it,
As I bide my time to see.

There's no control apparent,
Observing all can do.
The strangest sense is present,
As I wait for signs of You.

A visit not expected,
A thought for jester farm.
If it had occurred to me,
Be left with much alarm.

Your presence is more subtle,
A wisp that's hardly noted.
You manifest as Goodness,
To that I am devoted.

So holding and observing,
Is all that I can do.
Keeping the suggestion
Quiet and subdued.

It seems when there is synchrony,
Your Hand may be suspected.
But then there's chance or randomness,
More than what's expected.

Still I wait with hopefulness,
No doubt does cross my mind.
Reflecting over lifetime,
The sense of You I find.

Perhaps that's all You'll offer,
A game to not be played.
The blessings of Your Grace and Love
Is all you need to say.

Clarity

I suspect I've missed a point,
It's slow of me, forgive.
The concept of connecting,
Appears, for all we live.

Without it we are nothing,
No sense of self or life.
Even though when filled with it,
There's still no end of strife.

So what is the emotion,
We experience and breath?
The feeling of connection,
When lost we're left to grieve.

What is felt so tender,
At other times intense.
It seems so very obvious,
Defining existence.

Esteemed in all of poetry,
Revered in sacred script.
No end of recognising it,
From birth, beyond the crypt.

Connecting is allusion,
To a valued sense of care.
Reciprocal involvement,
The answer to despair.

Its hold creates security,
Lifts you to Above.
Of course, it is so obvious!
The blessing to know Love.